THE SECRET of PERFECT SKIN

DIY HOMEMADE NATURAL BEAUTY RECIPES

MEG GORDON

ISBN-13: 978-1979885225

ISBN-10: 1979885222

Disclaimer

The purpose of this book is to help you with your outer image. The information in this book is true and complete to the best of the author's knowledge. All recommendations are made without guarantee on the part of the author. The author disclaims any liability in connection with the use of this information.

About the Author

Meg Gordon has been studying many great things in her life. She finished hairdressing school with some cosmetology involved. Then life turned her to the business and finance field with some personal development in mind and body health. She has been studying the greatest masters in the field and applying their wisdom. Her biggest passion is to help people to achieve a better lifestyle by applying positive thinking and making better choices in their lives. She went through many paths in her life and she has tried many things in order to pass this information to you. Her techniques can be easily applied immediately into your health and beauty improvement strategy as long as you make a commitment on your side.

Table of Contents

INTRODUCTION

I have decided it's time to take a control of my own body and health.

More and more people are realizing that body health is very important, and if you don't pay full attention to it, it will decline rapidly. This means, you will have to spend more time and more money to fix it ASAP in order to become healthy again.

Remember, that if you feel young in your heart, you will feel young in your spirit and body.

The important thing to remember is SELF-ESTEEM. Your first step in your new life should be to change your attitude. For example, if you feel old, you will be old in your spirit and in your body; however, if you will feel young in your heart, you will slow down your aging by many years. Yes, sociology and psychology play a huge role in your body and in your mind! The first step in this process is to figure out what it is you are doing or thinking that is making you feel old. Your own thoughts and old beliefs brought from your parent's house are not working anymore. They make you useless. Unhappy! Your thoughts are energies that support you in your day-to-day life. A good thought equals a better life. Bad, negative thoughts equal a bad life, bad habits, and bad self-esteem.

The second step after figuring the first step is to take control of your good thoughts. When you learn how to appreciate your thoughts, your mind will start doing amazing things. You will feel better, you will have more energy and you will have more aspirations. Aspirations are wonderful things. You might want to change your look and visit a hairdresser or go shopping for a new wardrobe. When new things appear in your life, you will find yourself more alive, vibrant and joyous. People will start noticing your new image. Therefore, go and celebrate yourself. Pay yourself first. You can do it by having a nice face mask, a body scrub, a manicure or take care of your hair. Those small things will build up and over time, you will find that you feel better. You have changed into a better and happier you.

Let your imagination run wild.

Choose your own schedule that suits you best.

Remember, stop staring at the mirror and stop looking at your wrinkles.

What you can notice by looking in the mirror is not always a happy image of yourself. The appearance of your wrinkles may make you feel down and depressed. There are many good face masks and scrubs, which I will introduce to you in the next pages. Those five-minute mixtures will help you take care of your skin and give you a better appearance. Those formulas are based on natural ingredients and will not cost you a bunch. The only thing you have to put into it is your time and your willingness to feel and look healthier. Trust me, it works on me, so it will work on you too.

Wrinkles appear not only on your face but also on the rest of your body. It is the natural way of aging, which we can't omit, but we can slow it down or prevent it.

A few more important factors, which you should take under consideration to change, include the following:

1. Appreciate yourself! In order to do this, write on a piece of paper your merits and abilities. This list should hang in a prominent place, e.g., on the mirror or refrigerator, so you can read it every morning or as often as possible. It is very important that you see yourself as worthy and important.

2. Do not worry about criticism. Be aware of the differences between argumentative and malicious comments. Please note that you consider the most negative comments from relatives, although you do not deserve them. Usually, this is due to their complexes. Remember that you are building self-esteem based on what you think about yourself and not based on what others say or think.

3. Believe that you deserve a lot. Thinking, "I'll never meet a nice guy or a girl, because I do not deserve it" is unfair and hurts you. Remember, you are entitled to have happiness, to be loved and accepted.

4. Accept yourself! Tell yourself, "I have advantages and disadvantages. I can't manage everything, but that's normal. I like myself, and I want others to like me for who I am.

5. The most important thing most of us forget is that Mother Nature provides us with many great things that are full of vitamins and minerals that can be used on a daily basis.

So, let's go on our journey of having lots of fun with them.

Face: Rejuvenation Mask

3 tablespoons natural yogurt

1 tablespoon honey

1 egg yolk

1 teaspoon lemon juice

Mix the ingredients. Spread the mixture on the face and neck. Leave for 30 minutes. Wash the face and neck with a cotton ball soaked in milk. Use the water spray bottle to spray your face. Towel dry your face.

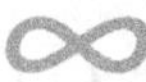

1 banana

1 avocado

2 tablespoon natural yogurt

1 liquid tablet of vitamin E

Mix the ingredients in a mixer. Spread the mixture on your face and neck for 20-30 minutes. Wash your face with lukewarm water.

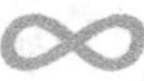

1 tablespoon honey

1 tablespoon fresh lemon juice

1 tablespoon olive oil

Mix the ingredients in the bowl. Spread the mixture on your face and neck for 10-20 minutes. Rinse with lukewarm water.

3 teaspoons raw oats

¼ teaspoon apple cider vinegar

1 teaspoon honey

1 drop tree oil or basil oil

Grinder the dry oats for smaller pieces. Add honey and apple cider vinegar. Mix till it is a smooth mixture. If you desire to add additional honey, you may do that. At the end, add 1 drop of tree oil or basil oil and mix it again.

Pre-wash your face; gently dry by patting with a towel. Apply the mixture and with a circular motion, massage it. Avoid the eye area. Leave it for 15-20 minutes. Wash off with lukewarm water.

NOTE: If you think you might have allergies towards essential oils, please perform a skin patch test before using any.

1 teaspoon clay/kaolin

1 teaspoon oats

1 teaspoon cornflower

1 egg white

1 teaspoon jojoba oil

1 drop chamomile oil

1 drop frankincense oil

1 drop myrrh oil

In a separate bowl, beat the egg white. Grind the oats into a powder.

Meg Gordon

Mix together all ingredients in a glass bowl. Apply this mixture on your face and gently massage it. Leave on for about 10-15 minutes. Rinse off with warm water. Repeat the process twice a week for best results. Apply moisturizer.

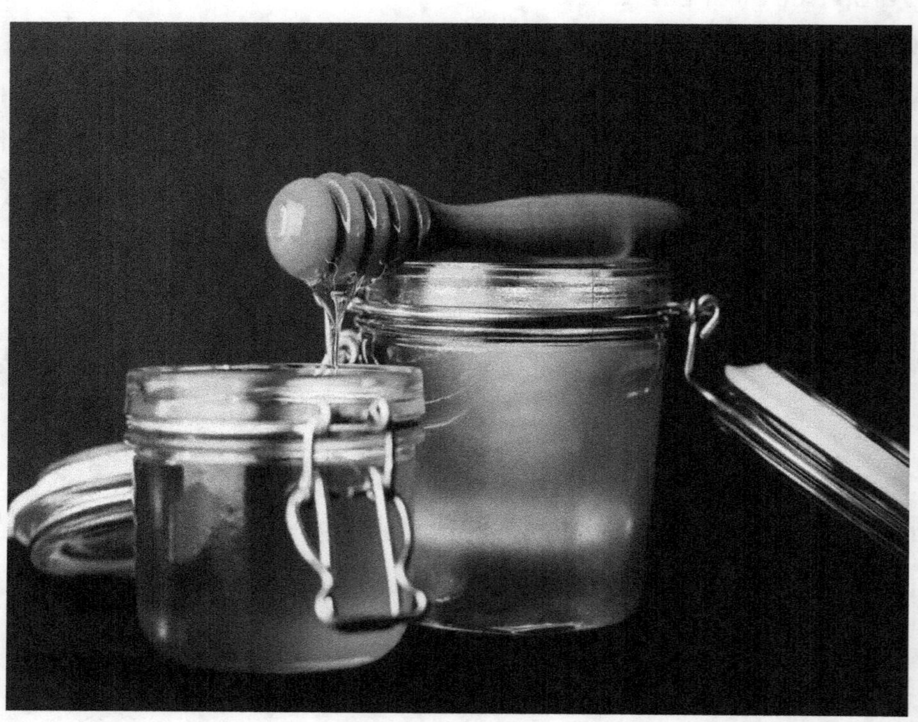

Face: Strengthening

5 tablespoons of oatmeal

½ cup boiled hot water

2 tablespoons plain yogurt

2 tablespoons honey

1 egg white

Combine 5 tablespoons of oatmeal with ½ cup of boiled hot water. Let it soak for 3-5 minutes. Add the rest of the ingredients and mix it all together. Apply it on a clean, pre-washed face. Leave it for about 15-20 minutes, then rinse off with lukewarm water.

Boil one potato without salt

1 tablespoon buttermilk

Mash potato and add the milk. Spread the mixture on the face. Leave it for 20 minutes. Wash your face with chamomile tea.

1 lemon (juice from it)

3 tablespoons olive oil

Mix it in a bowl. Apply on your face and massage thoroughly for about 5 minutes. Rinse off with warm water.

∞

1 tablespoon mayonnaise
Spread it all over your face and leave for 15-20 minutes. Wipe off with cotton balls then rinse with cool water.

1 ripe banana
Mash banana with a fork into a smooth paste. Spread it all over and massage gently in circular motion. Leave on for 15-20 minutes. Rinse your face with lukewarm water.

∞

Face: To Smooth Complexion/Tightening

1 egg yolk
1 tablespoon honey
2 tablespoons flour
Mix the ingredients into a paste. Spread the paste on face. After 20 minutes, wash off.

2 tablespoons baking soda
2 tablespoons water
Mix the ingredients into a paste. Apply on face and leave till it dries or about 15-20 minutes. Rinse off with cold water. Repeat this treatment as often as you wish.

½ fresh papaya
1 tablespoon rice flour
3 tablespoons honey
In a bowl, mash the papaya with a fork. Add flour and mix until you get a fine paste. At the end, add honey and stir it nicely.
Apply the mask on your face and neck. Massage gently with tapping. Leave it for about 20 minutes and rinse off with lukewarm water.

1 cup blueberries

2 tablespoons honey

Apply honey on your clean face. Blend blueberries in the blender for a smooth paste. Apply blueberry paste on your face by using plastic gloves (you don't want to have stains on your fingers). Leave the mask for about 30 minutes. Rinse off with lukewarm water. You might use any face cream if you desire.

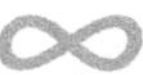

1 egg white

1 tablespoon aloe gel

Whisk the egg white first and then add aloe gel and continue whisking it smooth.

On a clean face, apply the mixture in an upward direction from chin up to your cheeks by using a brush. Leave till it dries. Use cotton balls dipped in water prior in order to remove the mask from your face.

∞

1 banana

½ cup whipping cream (could be sour cream)

Mash the banana in a bowl with a fork and add whipping cream.

Apply the mask on your pre-washed face and leave till it dries.

Rinse off with cold water and pat dry your face.

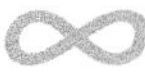

1 egg white

½ pre-chilled cucumber

1 teaspoon lemon juice

Blend the chilled cucumber in the blender first. Add egg white and lemon juice. Blend all ingredients once again.

On a clean face, apply the mixture in an upward direction from chin up to your cheeks by using a brush. Leave it for about 20-30 minutes. Rinse off with cold water and pat dry.

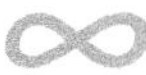

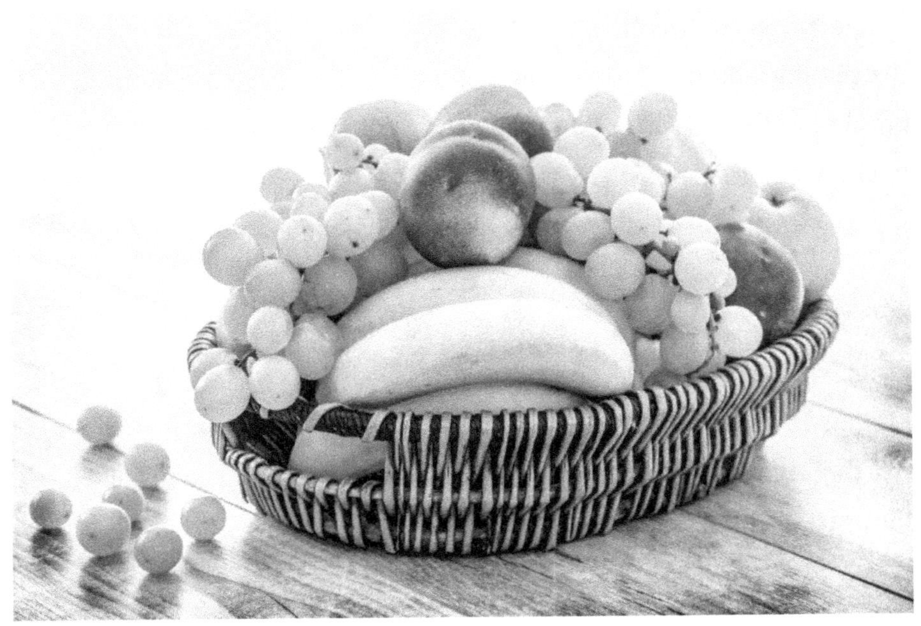

Face: Peeling

3 tablespoons oatmeal

5 tablespoons hot boiled water.

Mix the ingredients. When it cools off, you can spread the paste onto the face. Wash your face with lukewarm water.

2 peeled sour apples

Grate them and add:

2 tablespoons honey

2 tablespoons oatmeal

Mix the ingredients. Spread the mixture on the face. Leave for 10 – 15 minutes. When it dries, don't wash it off, just use your fingers and massage the masque.

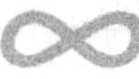

3 tablespoons sugar (white or brown)

3 tablespoons olive oil

Mix the ingredients. Spread the mixture on the face. Leave for 10 – 15 minutes. Rinse off with warm water.

1 tablespoon coffee grounds (you can take them from your coffee machine after you brew your morning coffee)

1 tablespoon olive oil

Mix in a bowl. Apply on your face and massage thoroughly for about 5 minutes. Rinse off with warm water.

You can use it every day as you wish.

2 tablespoons natural kefir.

Apply on your face and massage thoroughly. Leave for 10-15 minutes. Rinse off with warm water.

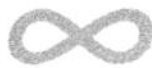

Face: Radiance Mask

1 fresh tomato flesh

½ peeled lemon

Mix the ingredients in a mixer. Spread the mixture on the face. Leave for 10-15 minutes. Wash your face with chamomile tea and apply your regular moisturizing cream.

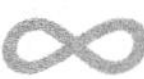

1 tablespoon plain yogurt

1 tablespoon honey

1 teaspoon lemon juice

Mix all ingredients in a bowl. Apply this mixture on your face and gently massage it. Leave it on for 5-15 minutes. Rinse off with warm water. Repeat the process 3-4 times a week for best results.

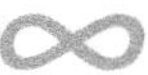

1 teaspoon honey

½ teaspoon baking soda

Mix all ingredients in a bowl. Apply this mixture on your face and gently massage it. Leave it on for 5-15 minutes. Rinse off with warm water.

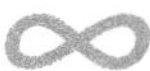

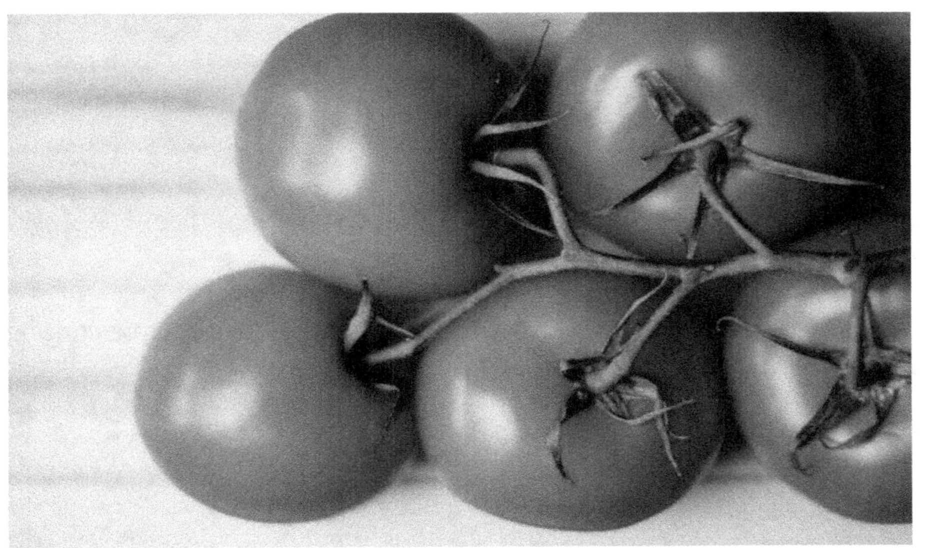

Face: For Tinting Effect

Grate 1 carrot

Add ½ teaspoon olive oil

Mix in a bowl. Wear plastic gloves on your hands to protect from tinting. Spread the mask on face for 15 minutes. Rinse off with warm water and finish off with tonic water.

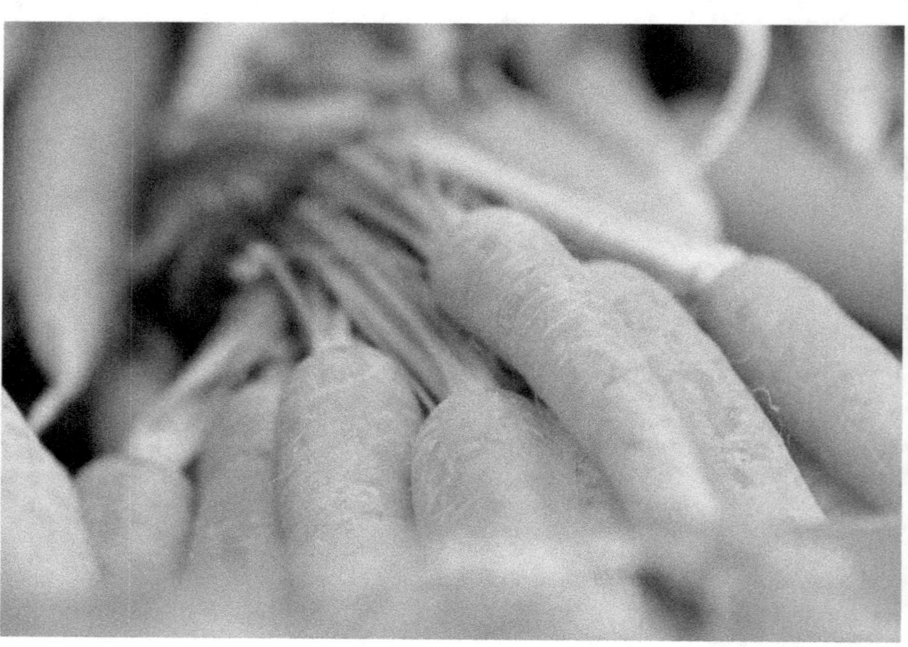

Face: Skin Blemishes and Wrinkles

Fresh (cream-like) royal jelly

Take a small amount of fresh royal jelly, apply on the skin at bed time, and massage the area every day for at least 4 weeks.

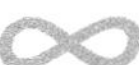

2 - 3 teaspoons of fresh lemon juice

1 teaspoon of honey

Mix them together. Apply on your face, emphasizing trouble areas (blemishes). Leave the mixture on your face for 5 minutes and then wash it with cold water. This mixture helps to fade marks/spots on the face and the honey will moisturize the skin.

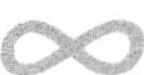

½ fresh cucumber

Grate it to a paste. Apply on your face, emphasizing trouble areas (blemishes/pimples/wrinkles or dry skin). Leave the mixture on your face for 20 minutes and then wash it with cold water.

½ fresh papaya

Smash the papaya with a fork. Apply on your face. Leave the mixture on your face for 20 minutes and then wash it with cold water. It helps reduce freckles or brown spots. For the best results, use this remedy for 7 days in a row.

1 tablespoon baking soda

2 tablespoons olive oil

Mix all ingredients in a bowl till you get a fine paste. Apply on your face and neck. Massage the skin for about 5-10 minutes in a circular motion. Wash off with lukewarm water.

Use it 2-3 times per week.

Face: Pimple or Acne

Take a garlic clove and cut the thick end into the square, but on the clove. Then take that cut edge garlic clove and press into a pimple. The juice from the garlic will cover your pimples.

Leave it overnight. Wash of the face in the morning. Your pimples should be gone.

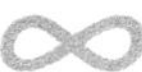

7 fresh strawberries

1 tablespoon sour cream

Mash fresh strawberries with a fork and then add sour cream.

Apply the mixture on clean, pre-washed face and leave it for 10-15 minutes. Wash the face with warm water. Use the mask twice a week for next 4 consecutive weeks.

½ teaspoon cinnamon powder

½ teaspoon honey

Mix ingredients together. Apply to blemishes and leave on your face for 20 minutes. Then wash it off with warm water.

Meg Gordon

1 banana peel

Rub the banana peel on the affected area (acne) for a few minutes until the inside of the peel turns brown. Leave it on for about 30 minutes. Wash it off with warm water.

2 tablespoons crushed burdock root

1 ½ glass water.

Take a medium cooking pot and add burdock root and water. Let the root absorb some water for approximately 30 minutes. Then, cook on medium heat for about 5 minutes. Leave the concoction under the cover for another 15-20 minutes. Strain the residue into a bottle.

Then take a cotton ball and pre-soak it into the solution; wipe your face 3 times per day.

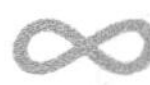

Face: Blackheads

1 teaspoon cinnamon powder

1 teaspoon honey

Mix it to form a thick paste. Apply the paste on the affected area before bedtime and leave it overnight. In the morning, wash face with water. For the best results, use this remedy for 10 days.

1 teaspoon cinnamon powder

1 teaspoon honey

1 teaspoon lemon juice

A pinch of turmeric powder

Mix it to form a thick paste. Apply the paste on the affected area before bedtime. Leave it for 20 minutes. Wash face with water. Repeat for 10 days.

(Please remember that turmeric powder may color your skin. Use brush in order to apply on your face.)

Meg Gordon

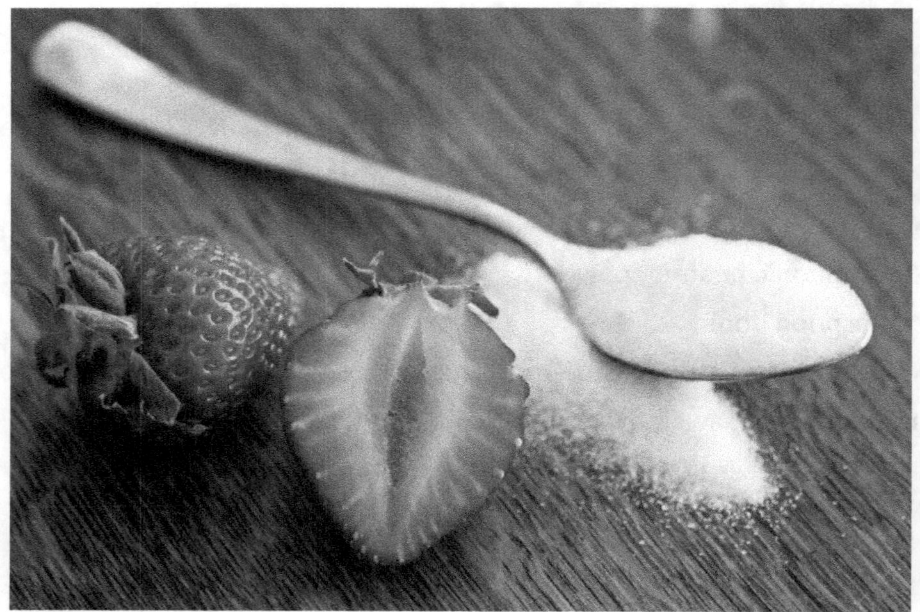

Face: Masque for Oily Skin

1 spoon baker's yeast

1 glass warm milk

Mix the ingredients. Then add:

1 spoon 3% hydrogen peroxide

Mix it again. Apply on the face. Leave till fully dry. Wash it with warm water then after with cold water.

2 egg whites

Whip the egg whites. Spread the egg whites on your face. Leave the masque till it dries. Wash your face with lukewarm water and apply tonic.

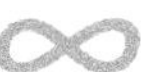

½ tablespoon turmeric

2 tablespoons oatmeal flour (could be also chickpea flour or kapha-barley flour)

½ teaspoon fresh lemon juice

¼ glass water

Mix all ingredients in a bowl. Apply to your face and neck. Massage for a minute or two. Wash your face with warm water or any herbal oils, e.g., coconut or almond oil.

Meg Gordon

You can use it every day if you wish.

Please keep in mind the natural yellow color of the turmeric might give you some natural tone. Therefore, it is recommended to use it prior to showering.

2 tablespoons baking soda

2 tablespoons water

Mix the ingredients into a paste. Apply on your face and leave till dry or about 15-20 minutes. Rinse off with cold water. Repeat this treatment as often as you wish.

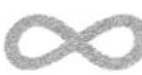

1 teaspoon clay/kaolin

1 teaspoon oats

1 teaspoon cornflower

1 egg white

2 drops rose water

1 drop lavender oil

1 drop juniper berry oil

In a separate bowl, beat the egg white. Grind the oats into powder. Mix together all ingredients in a glass bowl. Apply this mixture on your face and gently massage it. Leave it on about 10-15 minutes. Rinse off with warm water. Repeat the process twice a week for best results.

Apply moisturizer.

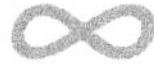

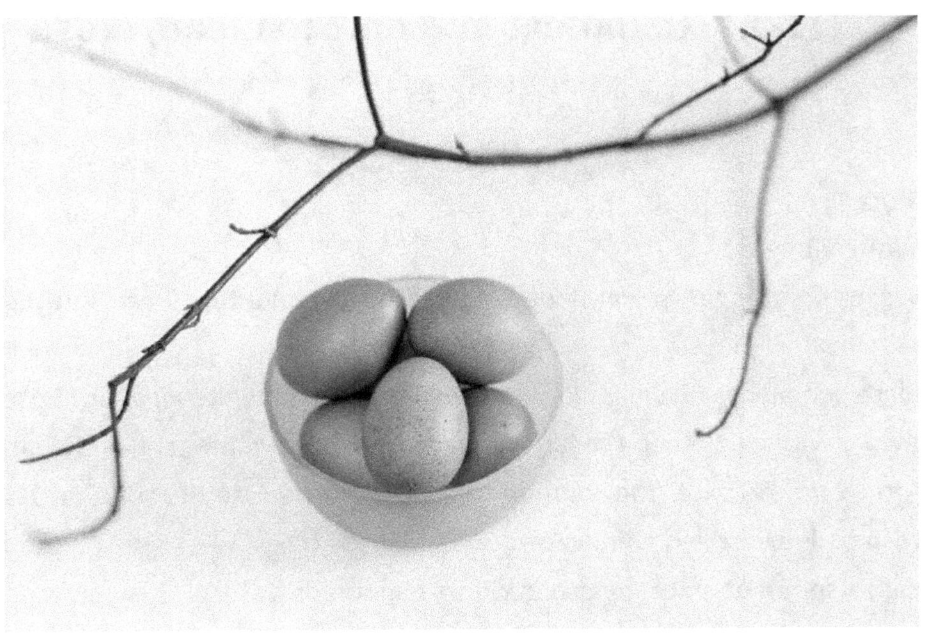

Face: Oily Complexion: Tonic to Clean/Close Pores

4 oranges

White vinegar

Wash the oranges in warm water. Peel the skin in a thin layer. Cut the skin in small pieces.

Place the pieces in a glass jar, and level them with white vinegar. Close the jar with a lid. Keep the jar in a warm place. Every day, shake the jar. After 2 weeks, filter the solution to a clean bottle. Use the solution 1:1 with boiled/distilled cold water.

E.g., 1 spoon of an orange solution to 1 spoon of water.

Use the cotton pads to clean your pre-washed face.

15 tablespoons lukewarm water

½ lemon juice

½ orange juice

Mix the ingredients. Wash your face with the tonic before bedtime. Keep the rest of the tonic in the fridge.

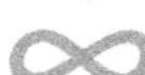

Few tulsi leaves (also known as holy basil)

½ cup hot water

Mix the ingredients. Leave covered for 30 minutes. Strain mixture and add 1 tablespoon aloe vera gel.

Apply this mixture on your face. Massage your face for about 10 minutes. Then leave it on for about 15 minutes. Wash your face with warm water.

Face: Oily Complexion to Close Pores

2 egg whites

½ teaspoon fresh lemon juice.

Beat the egg whites and add a lemon juice. Mix together. Apply to your face. Leave on till it dries. Rinse off the mask with cold water.

2 tablespoons water

2 tablespoons baking soda

Mix the ingredients in a bowl. Apply the paste on your face and leave for about 15-20 min. Once the mask is dry, use cold water to rinse off. Repeat this for 5-7 days or as often you desire.

2 tablespoons baking soda

2 tablespoons water

Mix the ingredients into a paste. Apply on your face and leave it till dries or about 15-20 minutes. Rinse off with cold water. Repeat this treatment as often as you wish.

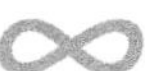

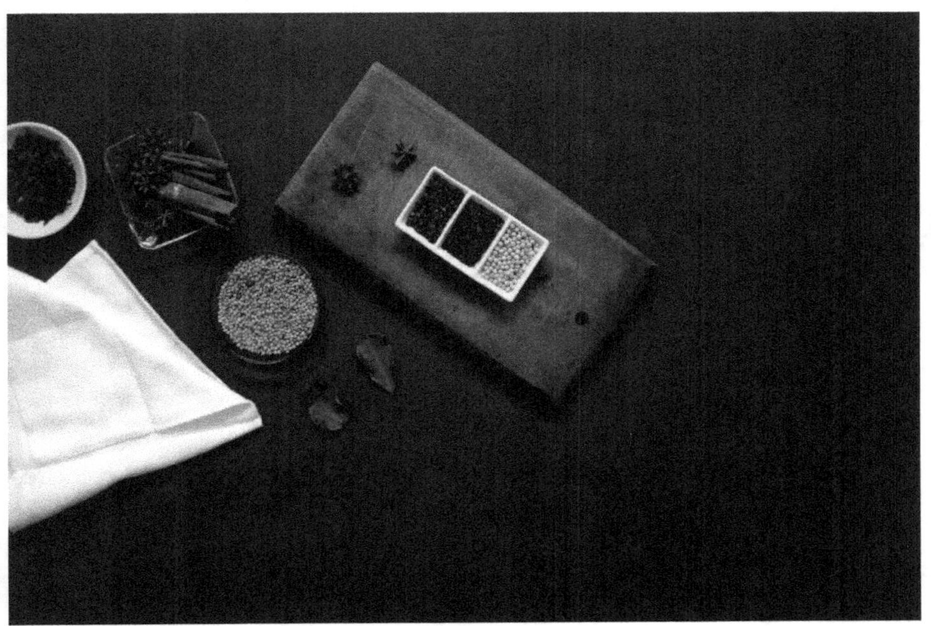

Face: Peeling for Oily Complexion

4 tablespoons baker's yeast

1 teaspoon honey

Add distilled water.

Mix the ingredients. It has to be thick in consistency.

Spread the masque on your face and neck. Keep it for 10-15 minutes.

Rinse off with warm water.

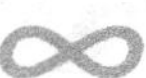

2 tablespoons cane sugar

2 tablespoons honey

2 tablespoons olive oil

1 teaspoon dried rosemary

5 drops lemon essential oil

5 drops lavender essential oil

Mix sugar, honey, olive oil and rosemary first. Then add essential oils. Apply this mixture on your face. Massage your face for about 2-3 minutes. Then leave it on for about 15 minutes. Wash your face with warm water.

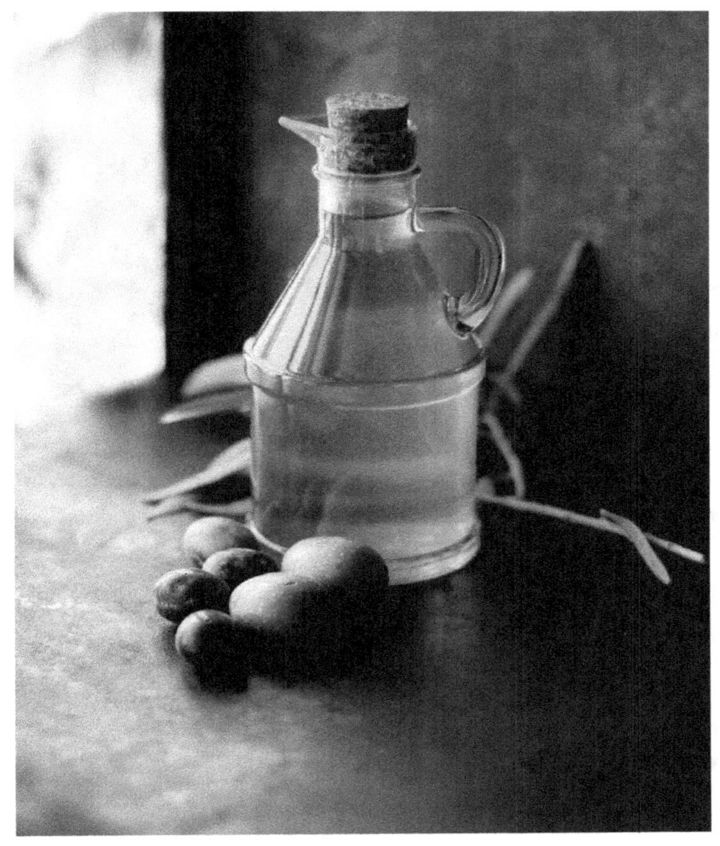

Face: Masque for Normal Skin

½ orange

1 tablespoon flour

1/3 glass of milk

Mix the ingredients into a paste. Spread the paste on the face and neck. Keep it for 30 minutes. Wash your face and neck with lukewarm boiled water. Repeat the treatment as often as you like.

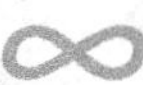

1 egg yolk

2 teaspoons honey

2 teaspoons wheat flour

Mix the ingredients into a paste. Spread the paste on the face and neck. Keep it for 20 minutes. Wash your face and neck with lukewarm boiled water. Repeat the treatment as often as you like.

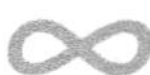

3-4 Aspirin tablets

1 tablespoon lukewarm water

1 tablespoon natural yogurt

Crush Aspirin tablets into fine powder, add water and yogurt. Mix it together. Spread the paste on the face. Keep it for 20 minutes and rinse off.

NOTE: If you think you might have allergies towards essential oils, please perform a skin patch test before using any.

1 teaspoon clay/kaolin

1 teaspoon oats

1 teaspoon cornflower

1 egg white

2 drops rose water

1 drop geranium oil

In a separate bowl, beat the egg white. Grind the oats into powder. Mix together all ingredients in a glass bowl. Apply this mixture on your face and gently massage it. Leave for 10-15 minutes. Rinse off with warm water. Repeat the process twice a week for best results.

Apply moisturizer.

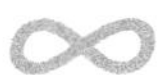

Face: Normal Complexion: Tonic to Clean/Smooth Complexion

1 cucumber

½ pre-boiled cold water

Peel off the cucumber and grate it. Add water. Mix together and leave the mixture for a few hours.

Strain the pulp. Use glass bottle in order to keep the liquid. Keep in refrigerator up to 3-4 days.

Use tonic twice a day as long as you wish.

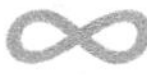

3 teaspoons water (boiled and cooled down)

1 teaspoon apple cider vinegar

Mix together. Wash your face and neck. Towel dry. Apply tonic by soaking a cotton ball in this toner. Use it every morning and night.

1 teaspoon sea salt

1 cup warm water

Take a clean bottle, fill it with sea salt and water. Shake well. Use it every morning and night after washing your face.

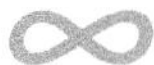

1 green tea bag

1 cup hot water.

Steep a tea bag in a cup of hot water for about one hour. Remove the tea bag. Pour green tea solution into bottle and keep it in the fridge. Use it every morning and night after washing your face.

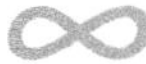

Face: Masque for Dry Skin

1 tablespoon orange juice

1 egg yolk

Mix ingredients into a paste. Spread the paste on the face and neck. Keep it for 30 minutes. Wash your face and neck with lukewarm boiled water. Repeat the treatment as often as you like.

½ teaspoon chickpea flour

½ teaspoon turmeric powder

½ teaspoon almond oil

½ teaspoon natural yogurt

Mix the ingredients into a paste. Spread the paste with a brush on a clean and dry face. Avoid eye area. Leave for 5-15 minutes. Wash your face and neck with lukewarm boiled water. Apply moisturizer or rose gold elixir.

1 egg yolk

1 teaspoon honey

1 teaspoon olive oil

1 tablespoon chamomile tea

Mix the ingredients in a bowl. Apply on clean, dry face. Leave for 10-20 minutes. Rinse off with warm water and apply moisturizer cream.

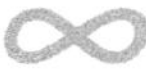

1 banana peel
1 cup coconut milk
Chop a banana peel in a blender and add coconut milk. Mix.
Apply to pre-washed face and leave for 20-30 minutes. Rinse off with warm water.

NOTE: If you think you might have allergies towards essential oils, please perform a skin patch test before using any.

1 teaspoon clay/kaolin
1 teaspoon oats
1 teaspoon cornflower
1 egg white
2 drops rose water
1 drop chamomile oil
2 drops carrot seed oil
In a separate bowl, beat the egg white. Grind the oats into powder. Mix together all ingredients in a glass bowl. Apply this mixture on your face and gently massage it. Leave for 10-15 minutes. Rinse off with warm water. Repeat the process twice a week for best results.
Apply moisturizer.

Meg Gordon

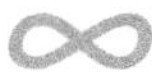

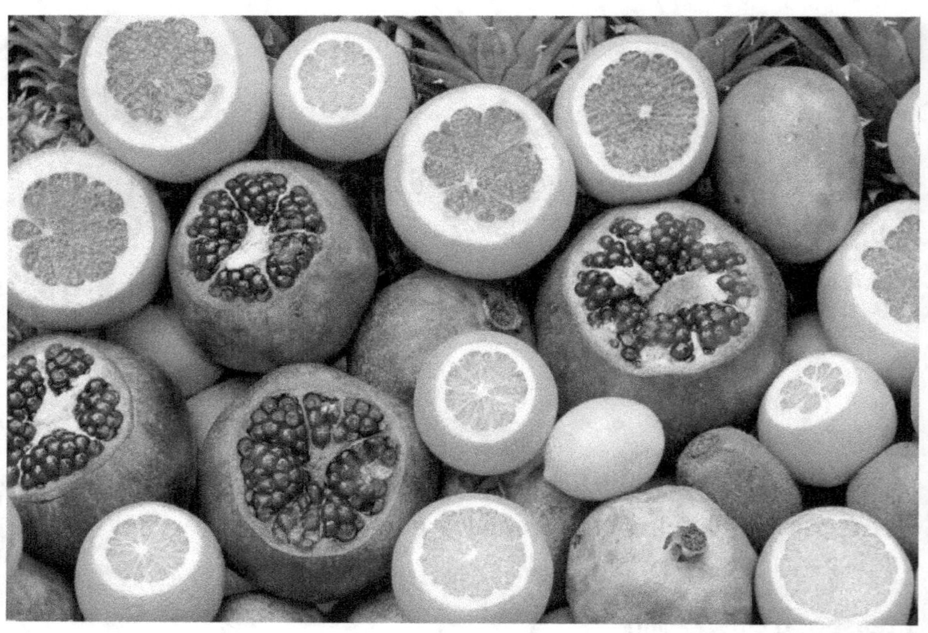

Face and Thorax: For 40+ or Extremely Dry Skin (e.g., after tanning)

½ glass sweet cream – whip it till stiff

1 teaspoon flour

Mix ingredients into a paste. Spread the paste on face and neck. Leave for 20 - 30 minutes. Wash face and neck with lukewarm boiled water. Repeat the treatment as often as you like.

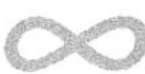

1 small box natural yogurt (100 ml)

1 tablespoon olive oil

Mix ingredients. Spread paste on the face or neck or thorax. Keep it for 10 - 20 minutes. Wash it off with lukewarm boiled water. Repeat the treatment as often as you like.

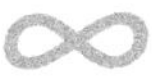

1 egg yolk

1 teaspoon honey

1 teaspoon olive oil

2 tablespoons strong brewed (chilled) chamomile tea

Mix ingredients. Spread paste on face or neck or thorax. Leave for 10 - 20 minutes. Wash it off with lukewarm boiled water. Repeat the treatment as often as you like.

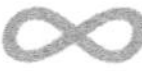

1 teaspoon honey

A few drops fresh lemon juice

A few drops sweet almond oil

Mix ingredients. Apply to face or neck or thorax. Leave for 10 - 20 minutes.

Rinse off with warm water.

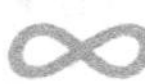

5 tablespoons organic carrot juice

1 tablespoon cornstarch

1 tablespoon sour cream

100 ml water

In a cooking pot, mix 100 ml of water with cornstarch. Put it to boil on medium heat. Stir the mixture until it thickens. Leave the pot on the side till it cools. Add carrot juice and sour cream. Mix all together for a nice paste.

Wash your face, towel dry. Apply the paste and leave for 30 minutes. Rinse with warm water.

Please note, the remaining mixture can be store in the fridge and used next time. For best results, apply 3 to 5 times per week.

1 garlic clove

1 teaspoon honey

1 tablespoon clay powder

Mash the garlic nicely then add honey and clay powder. Stir the mixture.

Apply to your clean face and neck and leave for about 20-30 minutes.

Rinse off with warm water.

Repeat it every day for 7 days.

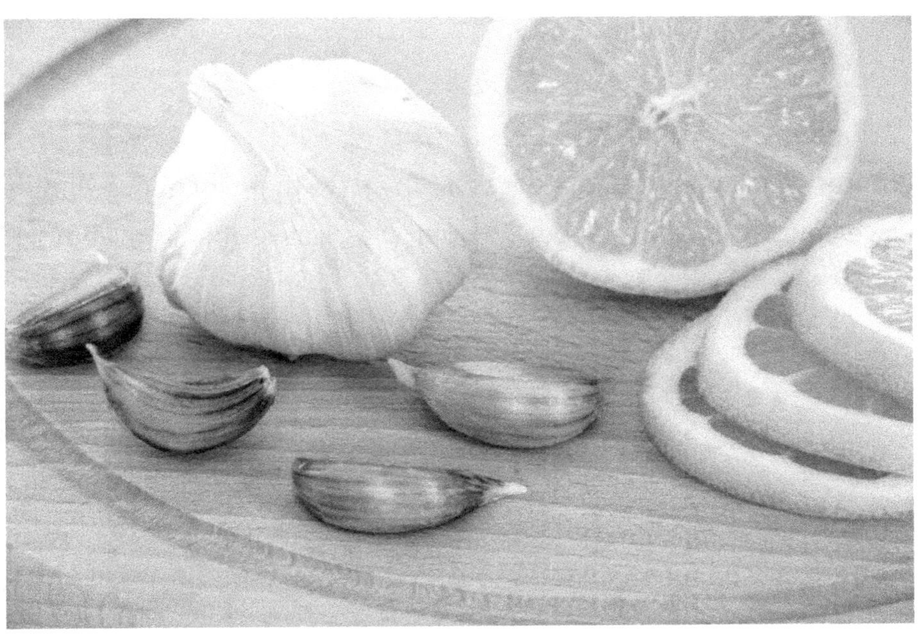

Face: Dark Circles under the Eyes or Puffy Eyes

Potato juice

Soak cotton balls in potato juice (fresh) and apply on your eyelids and on area under your eyes. Leave the cotton balls for about 15 minutes. Rinse off with warm water.

Cucumber

Cut fresh cucumber into thin slices. Refrigerate them for about 2 hours. Place cold slices of cucumber on your eyes. Leave them for about 15 minutes.

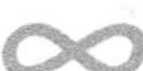

Tea Bags

Brew two tea bags in a cup for 5 – 10 minutes. Place each tea bag on your eyes for about 15 minutes to get relief from dark circles and puffy eyes. Remove them and rinse off with warm water.

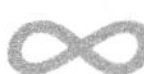

Apple cider vinegar (ACV)

Soak a cotton ball in ACV. Massage gently under your eyes in a circular motion for about 5 minutes. Rinse off with warm water. You may apply

ACV twice a day for better results.

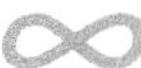

Coconut oil

Take a few drops of coconut oil onto your fingers and gently massage around your eyes in a circular motion for about 5 minutes. If you need to clean your eyes of too much access oil, you can just wipe off with a cotton ball. Repeat as often as you wish.

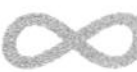

Cold compress

You can use anything that was chilled before in the freezer. For example: brewed tea bags, an ice bag, frozen meat. But please remember to wrap in a cloth before placing on your eye lids. Otherwise, you might get frostbite!

Rose water

Soak cotton balls in rose water and apply on your eyelids and on area under your eyes. Leave the cotton balls for about 15 minutes then remove the cotton from your eyelids. You might rinse off with warm water. Repeat it as often you wish.

Meg Gordon

Orange juice

2-3 tablespoons of orange juice

½ tablespoon glycerin

Mix ingredients. Soak a cotton ball in the solution. In a circular motion, gently massage skin around your eyes for 2-3 minutes. Remove the access with a dry cloth. Repeat as often as you wish.

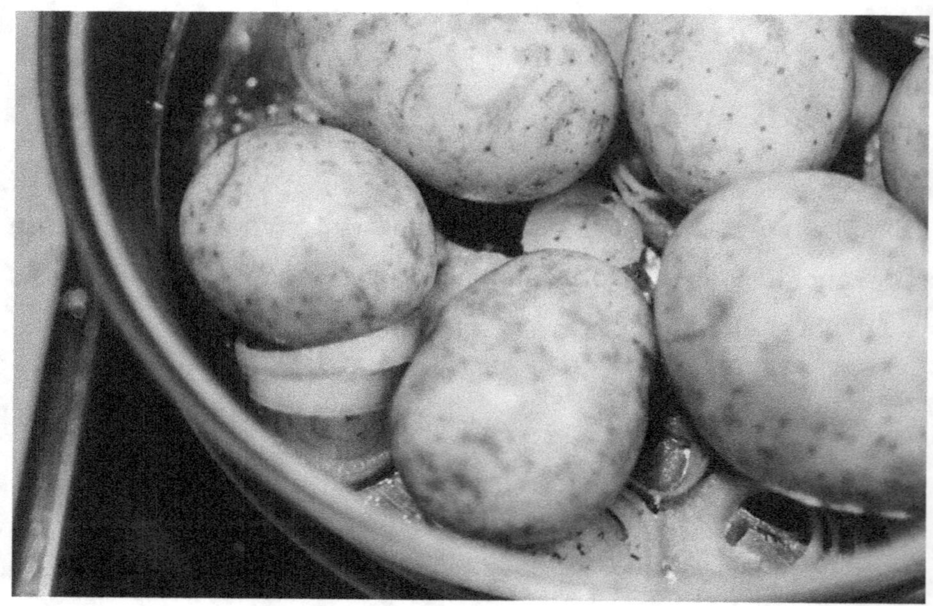

For Stronger and Healthier Hair (Prevents Getting Greasy Hair)

2 Black or white turnips/radishes
You can use a juicer in order to separate the pulp and juice. When you have juice ready, massage it gently into your scalp. Wrap it with the plastic wrap. Keep it for 2 hours. Wash your hair. Repeat this treatment once a week for 2-3 months.

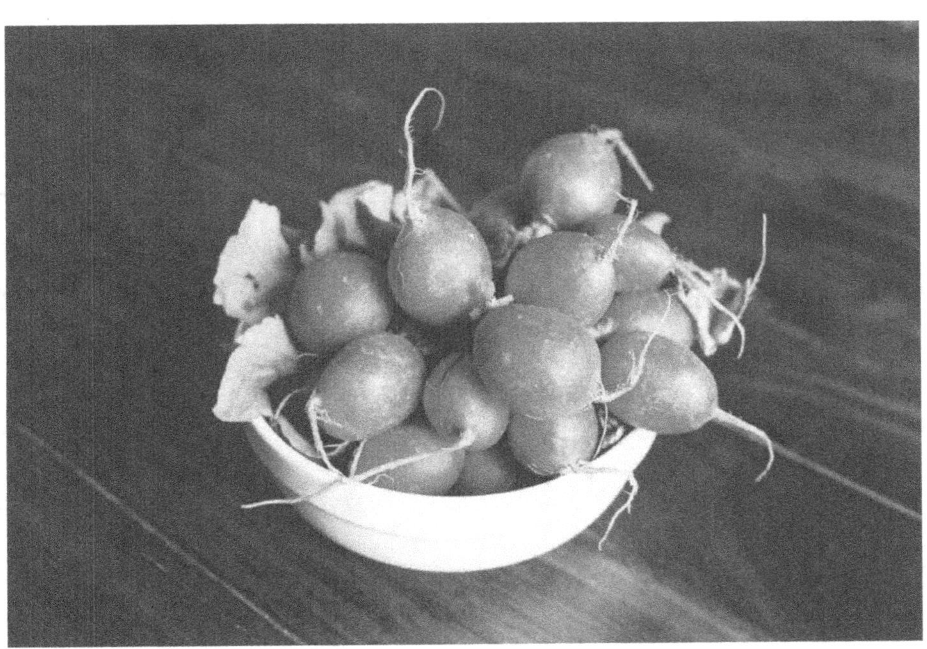

Masque/Rinse for Dry, Damaged, Brittle and Fine Hair

1 avocado

2 tablespoons sour cream

Mix ingredients in a bowl, wet your hair and towel dry. Put the mixture on your hair, massage the scalp and wrap it with plastic wrap. Leave for 30 min. Wash your hair.

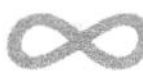

1 avocado

2 tablespoons olive oil

In a bowl, mix mashed avocado with olive oil until well combined. Wash your hair and towel dry. Apply the hair mask on the scalp and damp hair thoroughly. Tuck your hair in a shower cap and towel on top (to keep the heat). After 20 minutes, rinse off the hair mask while massaging the scalp. Shampoo as usual.

You can repeat it as often as you wish.

2 bags marigold tea

1 liter water

Boil the water and brew the tea for 15 min. Use the rinse twice a week after regular hair wash.

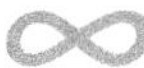

1 egg

3-4 tablespoons beer

Mix ingredients in a bowl; wet your hair and towel dry. Put the mixture on your scalp and hair, massage the scalp and wrap it with plastic wrap. Leave for 30 min. Wash your hair.

1 tablespoon honey

1 tablespoon apple vinegar

1 glass warm water

Mix ingredients; wash hair as normal. Use the mixture as a rinse; do not rinse the hair after.

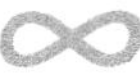

1 tablespoon olive oil

1 egg yolk

2-3 drops vitamin A

Mix ingredients; wash hair as normal. Put mixture on your scalp and hair; massage the scalp and wrap it with plastic wrap. Leave for 30 min. Rinse hair with few drops of lemon juice or white vinegar. Repeat the treatment every 2 weeks.

∞

100 grams honey

3 tablespoons olive oil

Mix the ingredients. Wet your hair in the mixture. Cover with a plastic cap. Leave for 30 min. Wash your hair as you normally do with shampoo and conditioner.

∞

2 teaspoons coconut oil

2 teaspoons honey

Warm it up till it becomes a liquid.

Then add

2 teaspoons plain yogurt

Mix all ingredients together

Apply it on your dry hair and work it through your hair. You might use a comb in order to distribute the masque better. Leave for 30 minutes. Wash it off.

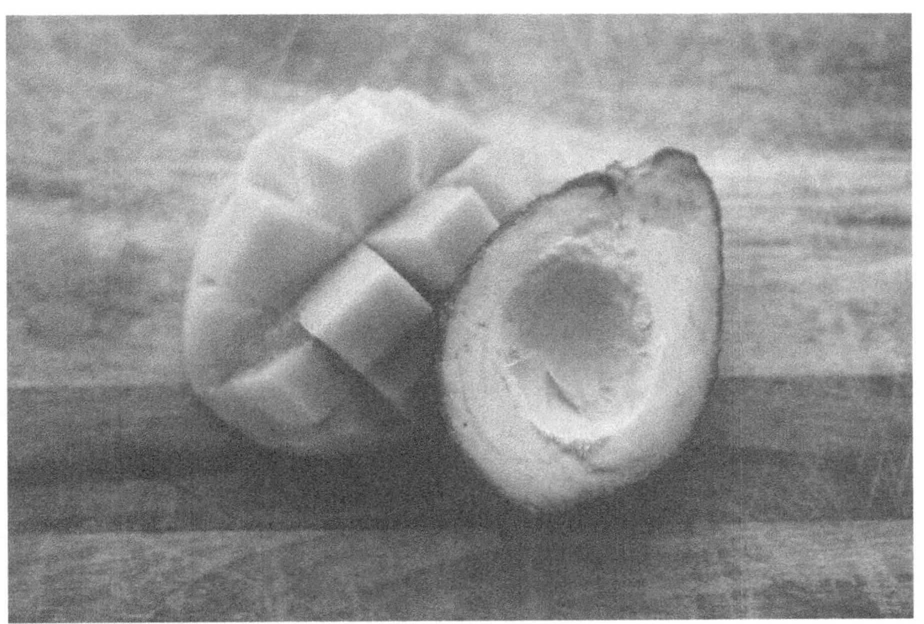

For Fine / Weak / Hair Loss / Dandruff

2 tablespoons horsetail (you can buy it at any health food store)

2 tablespoons Mydlnica Medical (Saponaria Officinalis)

2 tablespoons burdock

1 liter water

Brew the herbs for about an hour on low temperature. Shampoo your hair as normal. Rinse the scalp and hair with the herb solution. Repeat it every time after shampooing.

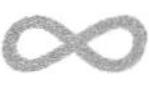

1 tablespoon baker's yeast

½ glass brewed chamomile tea

Mix it. Spread the paste on the scalp. Leave it for 30 minutes. Wash your hair.

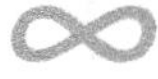

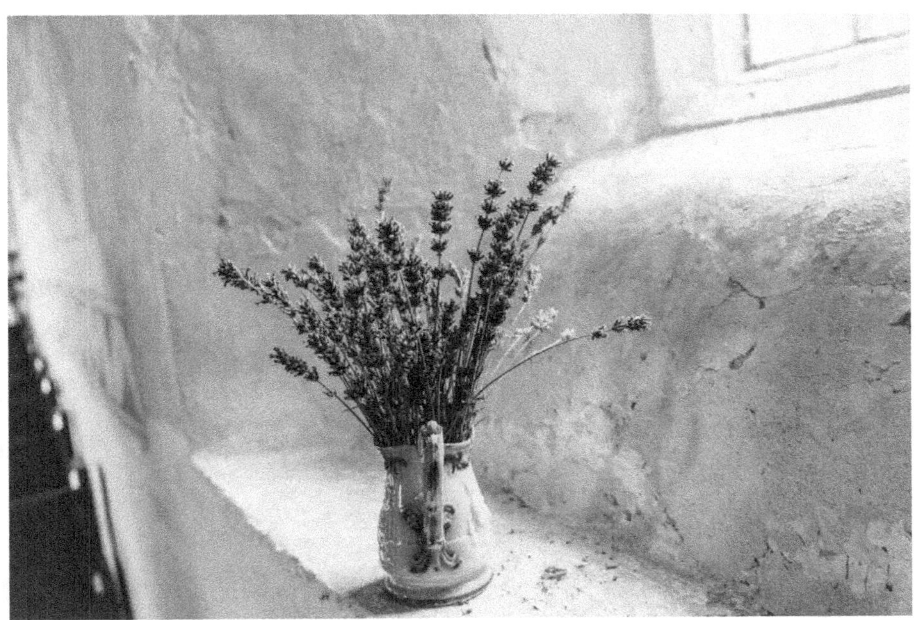

Dandruff

Coconut oil: On dry scalp, apply coconut oil and rub it into skin. Gently massage your scalp. Use shower cap and leave for 15-30 minutes. Wash your hair afterward. Repeat this at least 2 times per week. In winter time, you can do it more often.

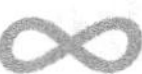

2 tablespoons olive oil

1 tablespoon almond oil

Mix the ingredients in a bowl. Apply this mixture on your scalp and hair. Massage your scalp and distribute the solution on your hair using a comb. Leave for 15-20 minutes under the shower cap. Rinse thoroughly.

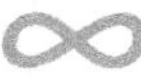

½ glass apple cider vinegar

½ glass water

Mix in a bottle. Apply the solution on your scalp and hair. Leave overnight. (You can use a shower cap or towel in order to keep your hair tight.) Wash it off and shampoo your hair.

Please note: If you have sensitive skin, use 3-4 times more water in preparation of this mixture.

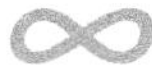

1 banana

½ glass apple cider vinegar

¼ glass water

1 teaspoon olive oil

Mix all ingredients in a bowl. Apply the paste on your scalp and hair. Massage your scalp for 5-10 minutes. Leave the mask for 20 minutes. Rinse/shampoo your hair. Repeat every day for a week.

Masque for Dry/Brittle Ends

1 egg yolk

3 drops lavender essential oil

Mix. Spread the paste on the hair ends. Wrap it with the plastic wrap. Keep it for 20-30 minutes. Wash your hair with shampoo. Repeat the treatment twice a week for 2-3 months.

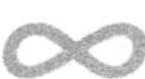

2 avocados

1 tablespoon olive oil

Mix ingredients into a paste. Spread the paste on hair ends. Wrap with plastic wrap. Leave for 20-30 minutes. Wash your hair with shampoo. Repeat the treatment as often as you like.

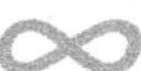

1 tablespoon chamomile tea

1 tablespoon nettle tea

1 tablespoon birch bark

½ glass boiled water

Brew the teas for about 15-20 minutes. Wait till it cools off. Strain. Add

1 egg yolk

1 tablespoon honey

1 lemon (add the squeezed juice)

2-4 drops essential rosemary oil

Then

Warm up a ¼ glass of olive oil and add all ingredients. Mix until smooth. Wash and towel dry your hair. Massage the masque into your scalp and hair. Leave for an hour. Rinse the hair with warm water. Repeat the treatment once a week for 2-3 months.

When Your Hair Is Getting Greasy too Fast

1 bag mint tea

1 bag nettle tea

1 bag chamomile tea

Few drops fresh squeezed lemon juice

Boil 3 glasses of water and brew the teas for 15 min. Use the rinse once or twice a week for 2-3 months after regular hair wash.

NOTE: Do not use it for highlighted hair, since it might cause a greenish cast.

½ long leaf aloe vera

½ glass warm water

1 teaspoon honey

Mix/chop the ingredients; wet hair. Massage the mixture into your scalp and hair. Wrap with plastic wrap for 20-30 min. Wash your hair as normal. Repeat the treatment every 10-14 days.

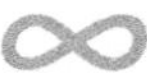

2 glasses nettle leaf

2 glasses boiled water

Brew until cold. Strain.

Add 1 glass 4% vinegar.

Mix the solution. Massage your scalp daily with the solution for 2 weeks.

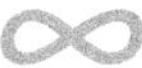

1 aloe vera leaf

Mix the leaf in the blender. Wash your hair. Towel dry. Massage the paste into your scalp. Wrap it with plastic wrap. Leave for 20-30 minutes. Rinse hair. Repeat this treatment after every shampoo for 2-3 weeks.

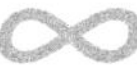

½ block baker's yeast (125 g)

½ glass milk

Mix ingredients. Massage into your scalp. Leave for 30 minutes. Wash hair. Repeat twice a week or as often as you would like to.

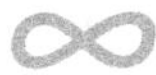

For Blond Hair / Fine Hair / Itchy Scalp

3-4 bags chamomile tea

1 liter boiling water

Brew the teas for about an hour on low temperature. Shampoo your hair as normal. Rinse scalp and hair with the chamomile solution. Repeat every time after your hair shampooing. The chamomile tea also highlights the hair.

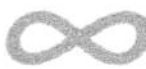

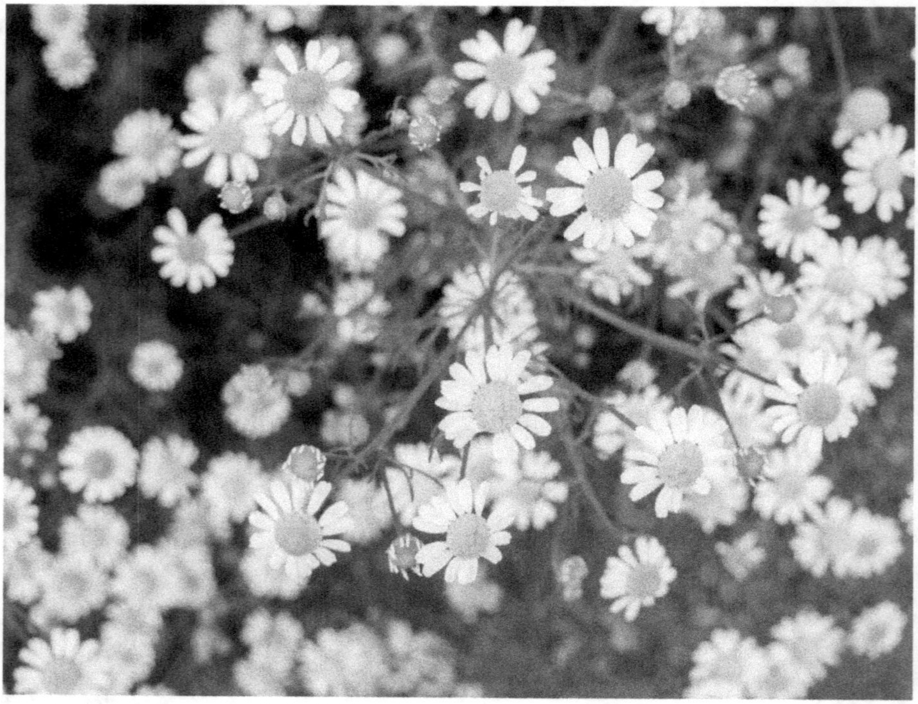

Tonic for Blond Hair

1 liter warm boiled water

1 teaspoon honey

1 lemon juice (1 lemon squeezed)

Mix ingredients. Wash hair as normal with shampoo and conditioner. For the final rinse, use the mixture prepared before. Rinse your hair and towel dry.

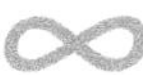

Peel 3 large parsley roots and boil them in 1 liter of water for 15 minutes. Wait till cool. Wash your hair with shampoo and rinse with water. Do not use conditioner; rinse hair with the pre-cooled solution. Do not forget to rub and massage your scalp gently.

Meg Gordon

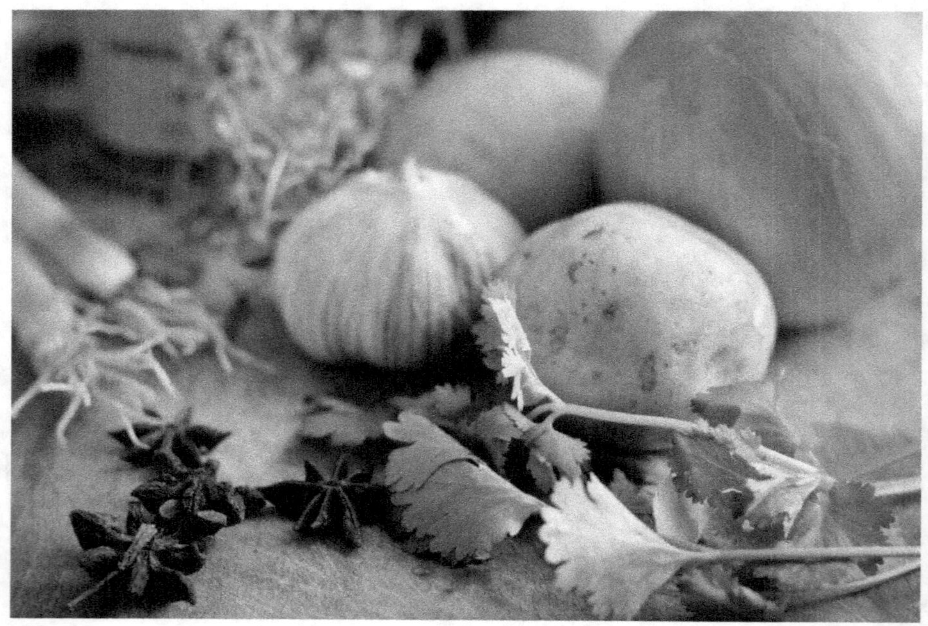

For Brown-Dull Hair

2 handfuls onion husk

1 liter water

Boil for 20 minutes. Wait till cool.

Pre-wash your hair. Dry your hair. Take the solution and rinse your hair. Make sure all is covered. Towel dry the excess solution. Proceed with blow drying your hair.

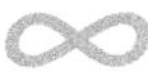

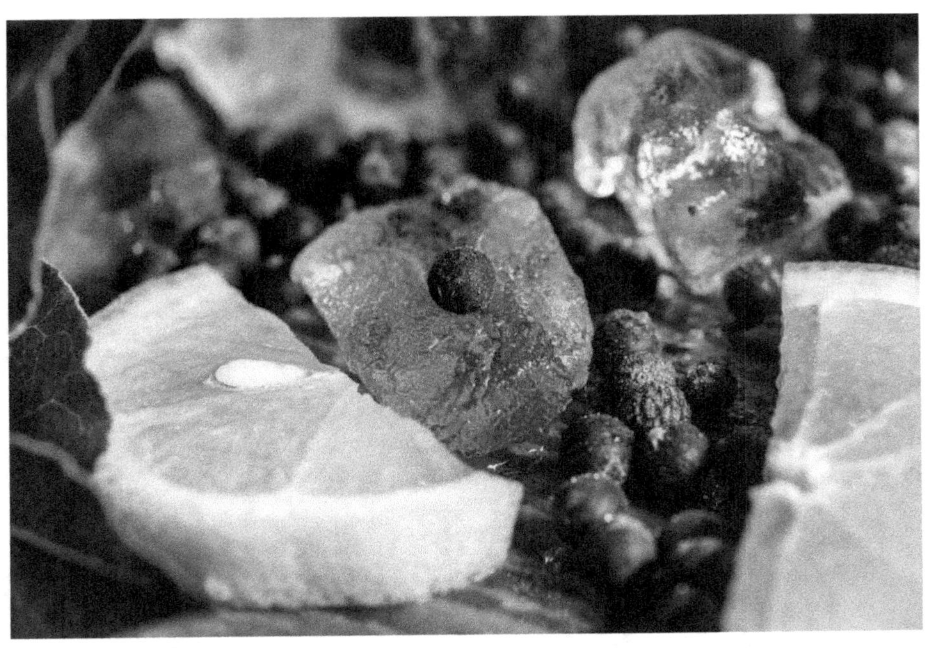

For Dark Hair

1 tablespoon black leafy tea

1 tablespoon sage tea

2 glasses boiling water

Cook it for 2 hours on mid-low heat. Add additional water in order to have the same level of solution in the cooking pot after evaporation. After 2 hours, cool it off and rinse your dry hair thoroughly. Wear a shower cap and wrap it with a warm towel. Leave it for 1 hour. Rinse off afterward.

∞

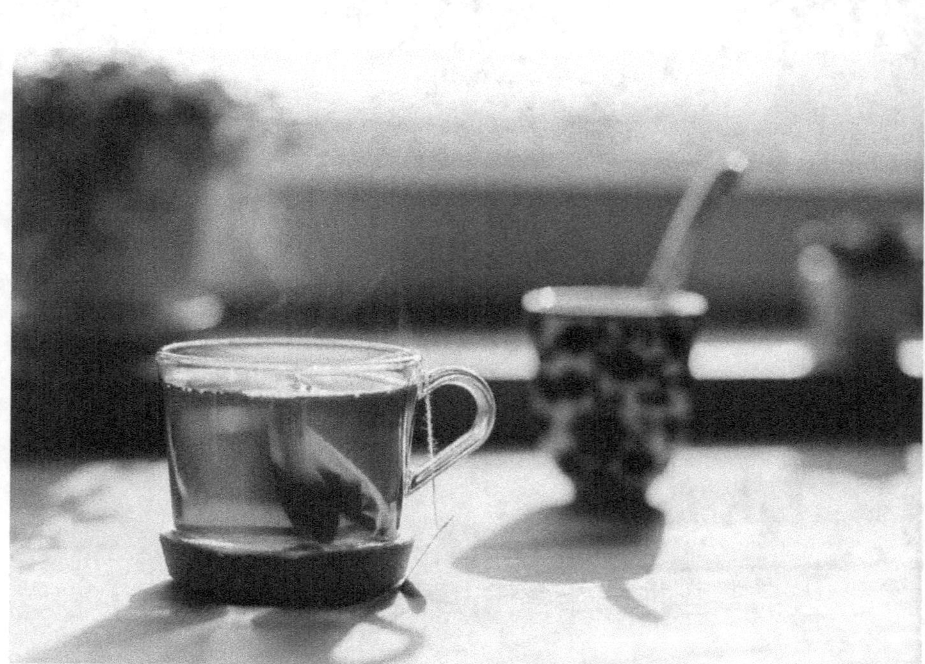

For Itchy Scalp

6-8 tablespoons buttermilk

6-8 tablespoons chamomile tea

Shampoo your hair as normal. Towel dry your hair. Massage the buttermilk or chamomile tea into your scalp. Leave for 15-20 minutes. Rinse hair with warm water. Repeat treatment once a week for 2-3 months.

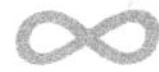

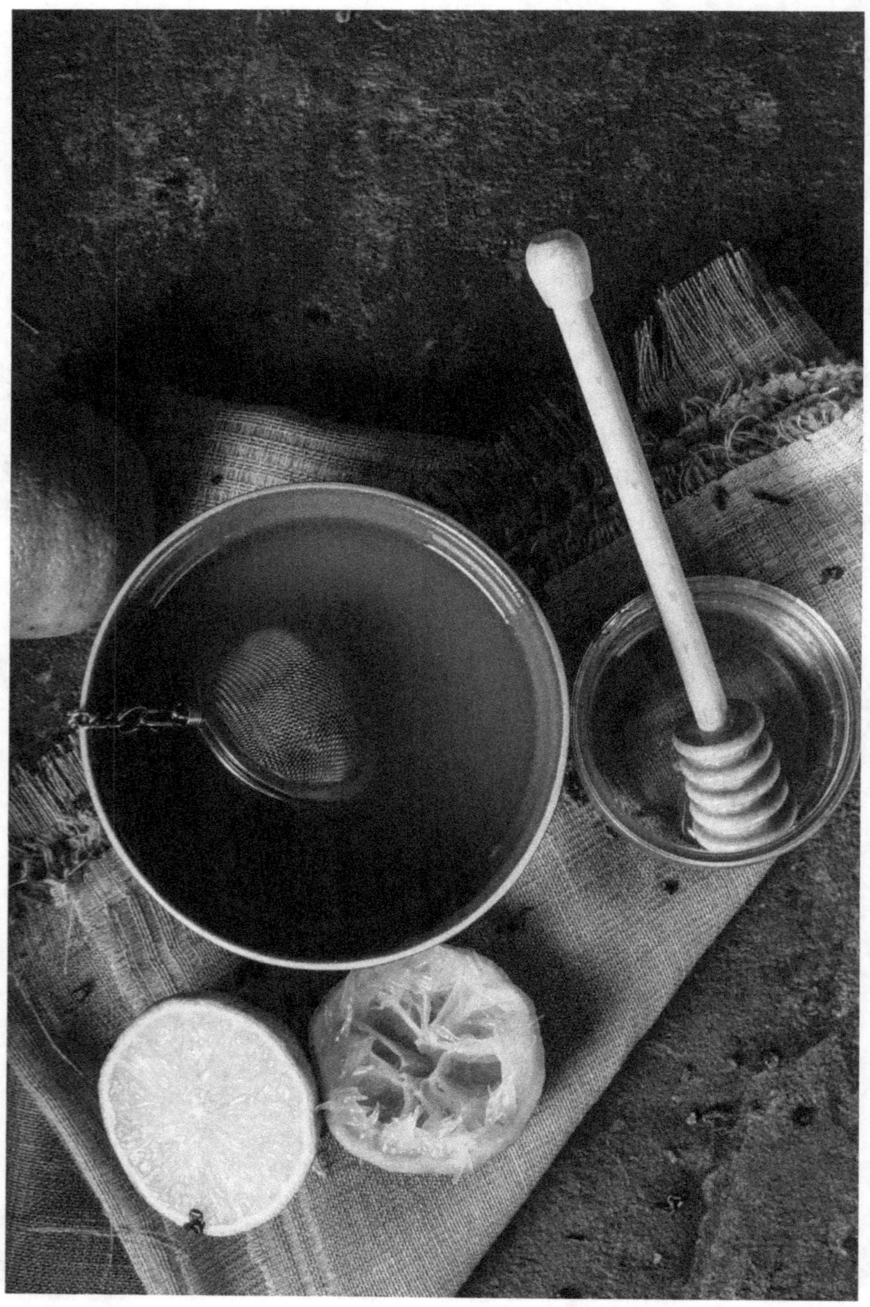

Natural Coverage to Cover Grey Hair

1 lb potato peels

2 cups water

In a cooking pot, boil potatoes. Stir and let simmer for about 5 minutes. Please make sure the pot is covered. After 5 minutes, remove from heat and let cool. When its cooled off completely, use the strainer in order to separate the water from the potato peels.

Shampoo your hair, towel dry and take a plastic cape and cover yourself. Take a hair brush and brush the water on your gray hair or use as a rinse. Make sure you use the potato water mostly on your gray hair.

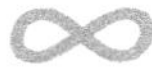

Masque Rinse (Lotion) for Colored Hair or Hair Loss

2-3 teaspoons castor oil (you can buy it at any pharmacy)

1 teaspoon fresh squeezed lemon juice

3 capsules vitamin B1

3 capsules vitamin B2

1 capsules vitamin C

Mix ingredients; wet hair. Massage the mixture into your scalp and hair; leave for 20 min. Wash your hair as normal with shampoo. Repeat the treatment every 2 weeks for 2-3 months.

2-3 tablespoons cosmetic kerosene

1 egg yolk

10 drops fresh squeezed lemon juice

10 drops castor oil

Mix ingredients; wet hair. Massage mixture into scalp. Wrap with plastic wrap. Leave for 20-30 minutes. Wash hair with shampoo. Repeat treatment twice a week for 2-3 months.

Grate the black radish and squeeze the juice from the pulp. Rub freshly made juice on dry scalp. (You will have a tingling sensation.) Wrap your hair with a towel. Rinse your scalp/hair after 30-45 minutes. Wash your hair with shampoo in order to rinse off the smell from the black radish.

50 ml distilled water

50 ml rosewater

15 ml apple cider vinegar

3 drops geranium oil

6 drops jojoba oil

5 drops rosemary oil

3 drops carrot oil

Mix all ingredients in a dark glass bottle. Shake the bottle every time before applying the solution into your scalp and then gently massage it. Leave it overnight. Shampoo your hair in the morning. Apply twice a week. Keep the solution in the fridge.

Rejuvenation Bath or Detoxify Bath

1 liter milk

3-4 tablespoons olive oil

Add them to warm water. Bathe in it for 15 minutes or longer. Repeat as often as you wish.

Prepare a bath with warm water. Add 300 g sea salt (coarse), add 1 glass of 12% coffee cream and 2 glasses of honey. Mix. Take a nice long bath for about 15-25 minutes. Afterward, rinse your body.

1 lb bag sea salt

1 box baking soda

Fill up a bath with warm water and mix the water with sea salt and baking soda. Sit in it for about 30 minutes, once or twice a week.

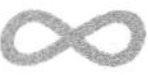

Bentonite clay pulls toxins out of pores, helps to heal skin, reduces redness.

Mix bentonite clay with warm water in a bowl. Apply on your skin in a circular motion. Wait till dry. Then rinse off with warm water.

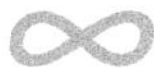

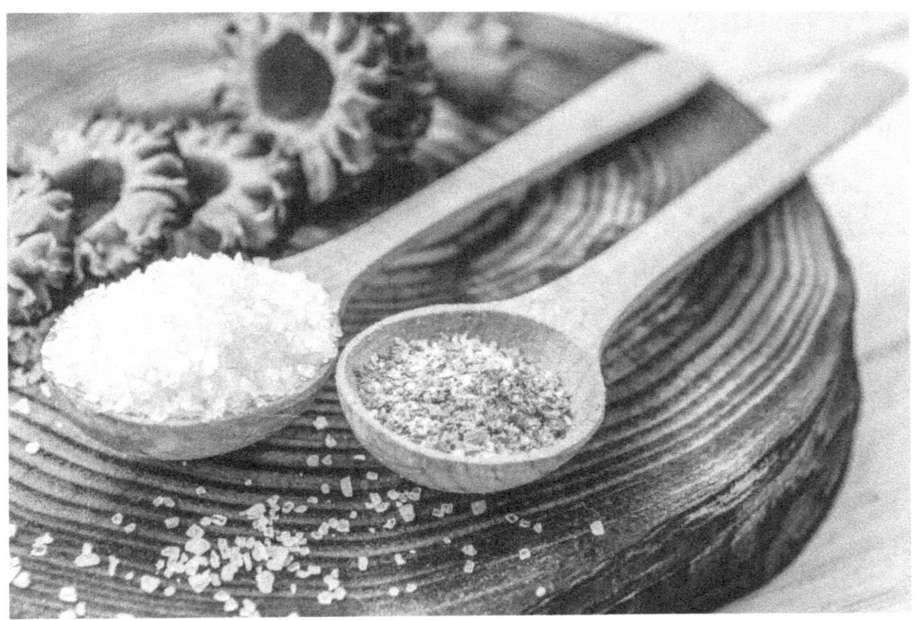

Body Peeling / Exfoliating Scrub

For this, we will need brewed coffee grained beans. (Basically, we recycle the coffee.)

So, take recycled brewed coffee and add shower gel. Mix in a bowl. Apply on your wet body and start applying it from your feet going upwards. You might use a loofah afterward to help you massage the body. Rinse off after 5 minutes.

3 tablespoons raw oats

2-3 tablespoons honey

1 tablespoon apple cider vinegar

1 drop of basil oil or tea tree oil

Grind the oats into a powder. Mix all ingredients in a glass bowl. Apply this mixture on your body and massage gently in a circular motion. Leave on for 5-10 minutes. Rinse with warm water. Repeat the process once a week for best results.

2 tablespoons honey

1 tablespoon lemon juice

3 tablespoons oats wheat

1 tablespoon coarse salt

½ glass olive oil

Mix all ingredients in a bowl. Apply and massage it on your body. Leave for 5-10 minutes and rinse off.

1 tablespoon sea salt

1 glass freshly made carrot juice

Mix freshly made carrot juice with sea salt in a bowl. Massage it on your scars in a circular motion or apply to any parts of the body. Leave to dry and rinse off with warm water.

Body Balms

Warm up a ½ glass of flax oil and massage it into your body. Leave for 30 minutes. DO NOT rinse off. Just use heated up towel in order to wipe up.

½ glass olive oil or flax oil

5 drops lavender oil

5 drops sandalwood oil

Mix ingredients in a bowl. Apply/massage it on your moist skin. Do not rinse off.

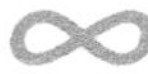

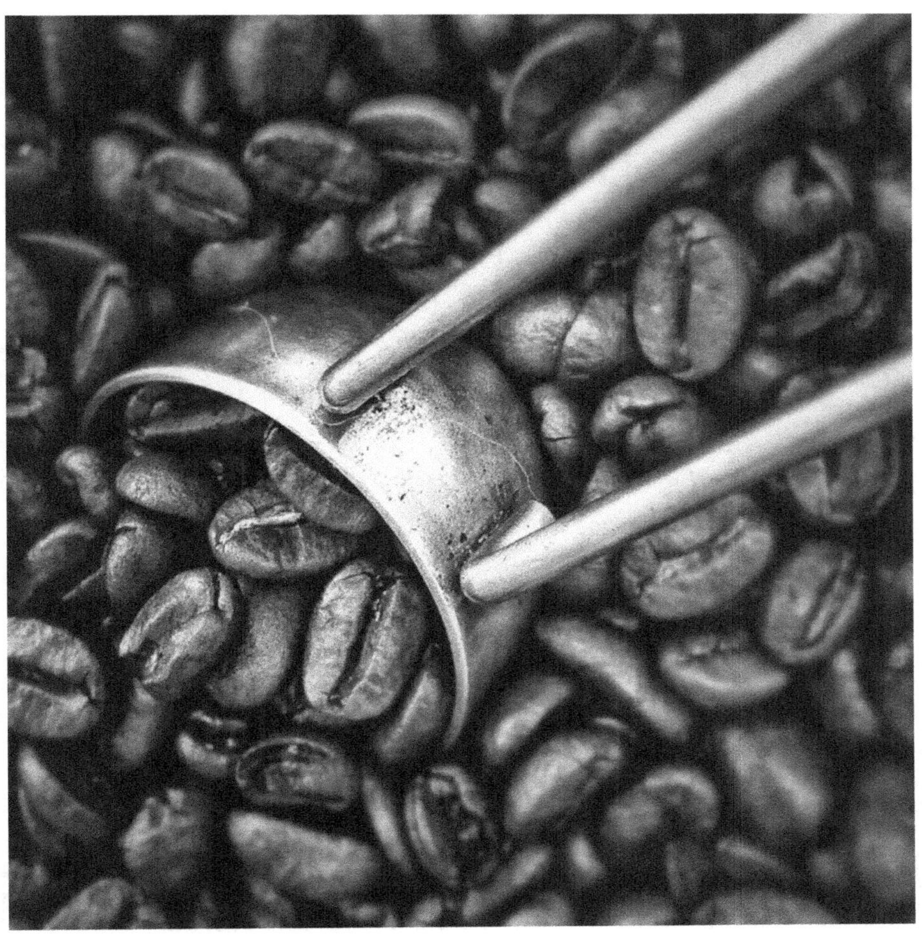

Hand Bath and Brittle Nails

2 tablespoons olive oil (warmed)

20 drops fresh squeezed lemon juice

10 drops vitamin E

10 drops vitamin A

Mix it and add warm water into the bowl. Keep your hands in the solution for 15-20 minutes.

1 tablespoon sour cream (18%)

1 teaspoon sugar

1 teaspoon fresh lemon juice

Mix all ingredients into a smooth paste. Apply on your hands for 5-10 minutes. Remove with a pre-oiled napkin with olive oil. Insert your hands into cotton gloves for 10 minutes. After that time, rinse your hands with lukewarm water.

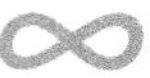

After boiling potatoes for dinner ...

Use the slightly warm potato water with a few drops of olive oil.

Sink your hands for 10-15 minutes. Repeat as often as you like.

2 tablespoons flax seeds

1 liter boiling water

Brew the flax seeds for 10-20 minutes, constantly stirring. When the water turns into a sticky liquid, then place on the side in order to cool down. When the solution is lukewarm, place your hands in it. Leave for 15 - 20 minutes. Repeat at least twice a week.

1 bag chamomile tea

½ cup buttermilk

Brew the chamomile tea. Wait till it is lukewarm, then add the buttermilk. Sink your hands in the bowl for 15 minutes.

NOTE:

After the hand bath, you can massage your hands with the additional masque. Wash it off after 10 minutes.

1 egg yolk

Few drops lemon juice

Mix the solution. Massage into your hands. Wash it off after 10 minutes.

Meg Gordon

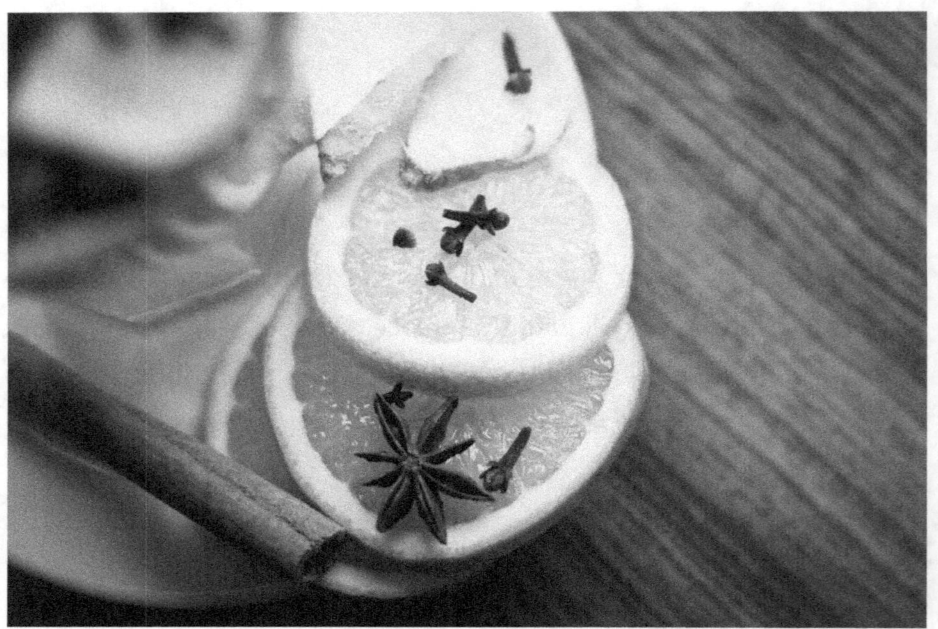

Brittle Nails

1 bag fennel tea (Foeniculi Fructus)

1 glass boiling water

Let it brew for 5-15 minutes. When the solution is lukewarm, take a cotton ball and dip into the solution. Then tap into nail beds 2-3 times daily. Use it daily for the next 3 weeks. (Brew your fresh fennel tea every 2 days.) You should see results after 3 weeks.

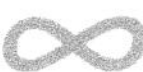

1 tablespoon castor oil

Warm it up and massage into your nails, cuticles, and hands. Repeat every 2-3 days.

1 tablespoon olive oil

½ teaspoon fresh lemon juice

Mix together in a small bowl. Apply the remedy on the nail, massage it and use cotton gloves. Leave it overnight. Use it twice a week.

1 teaspoon tea tree oil

Few drops vitamin E

Meg Gordon

Mix them together (you can store the rest in a small bottle). Massage the mixture on the nails. You can use it as often as you wish.

2 tablespoons sea salt

½ teaspoon fresh lemon juice

Few drops thyme oil

Few drops tea tree oil

Mix ingredients in a bowl and warm it up. Massage your nails and hands. Soak your hands for 15 minutes. Wipe with a towel. Repeat as often as you wish.

1 tablespoon olive oil

1 tablespoon apple cider vinegar

½ tablespoon beer

Mix all ingredients in a bowl and warm it up. Massage your nails and hands. Leave for 15 minutes. Rinse off with lukewarm water.

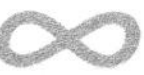

1 teaspoon coconut oil

Massage your nails and cuticles (you can use also on your hands as hand cream). Leave it. Do not rinse off. Use as often you wish.

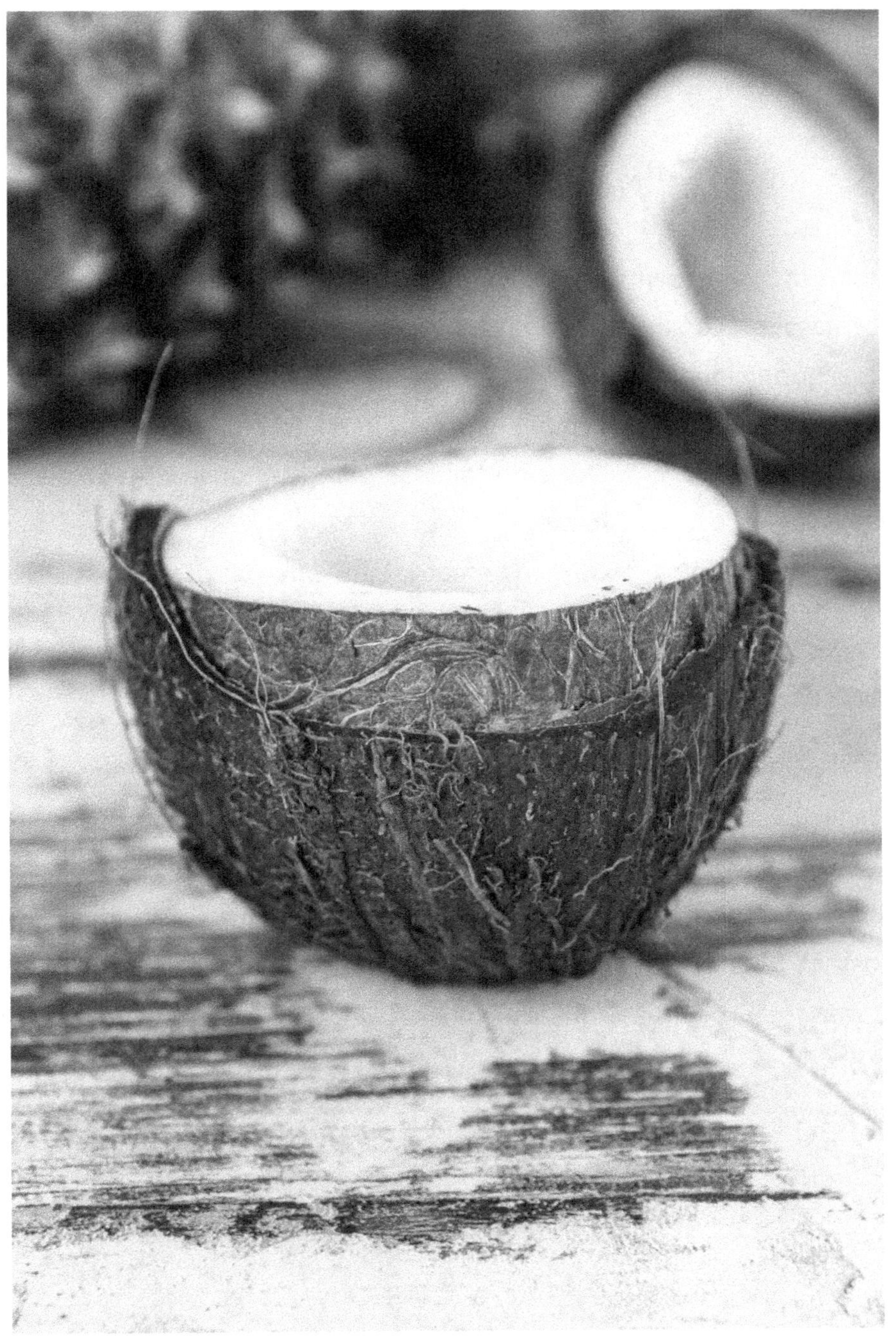

Beautiful and Youthful Hands

2 tablespoons brown sugar

1 tablespoon coconut oil or olive oil

1 teaspoon cinnamon

Mix all ingredients in a bowl. Apply this mixture on your hands and gently massage them. Leave on for 5-15 minutes. Rinse with lukewarm water. Towel dry your hands.

Keep the remaining mixture in a small jar and apply as often as you wish.

1 tablespoon plain yogurt

1 tablespoon honey

1 teaspoon lemon juice

Mix all ingredients in a bowl. Apply mixture on your hands and gently massage them. Leave on for 5-15 minutes. Rinse with warm water. Repeat the process 3-4 times a week for best results.

Cracked Heel or Red Skin

½ glass of sauerkraut

½ glass of boil potatoes water

Mix all ingredients in a bowl. Apply this mixture on your hands and gently massage them. Leave it on for 15 minutes. Rinse off with warm water. Apply greasy hand cream/Vaseline. Use cotton gloves. Repeat the process 3-4 times a week for best results at night time.

1 egg yolk

1 tablespoon olive oil

½ banana

Mix all ingredients in a bowl. Apply this mixture on your hands. Use plastic/nylon disposable gloves. Leave it on for 15 minutes. Use a cotton swab to gently remove the mixture from your hands.

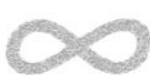

Meg Gordon

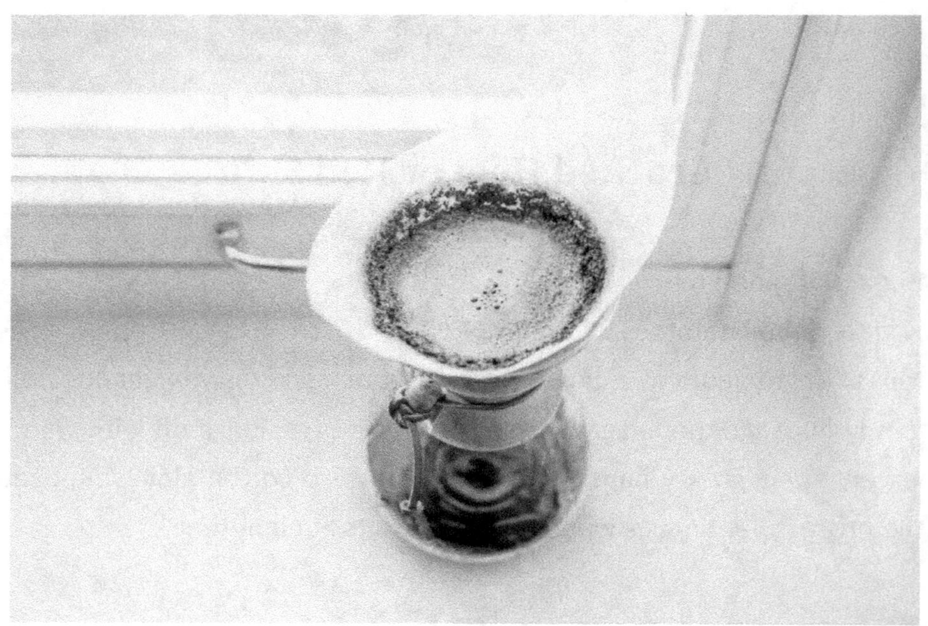

Teeth Whitening

For this type of teeth whitening, you will need a pair of latex gloves, a toothbrush and a metal sink (kitchen sink is good too). We need a metal sink because you will be able to remove the turmeric stains and from the ceramic one you will NOT.

½ teaspoon turmeric

½ teaspoon coconut oil

Few drops peppermint oil

Mix the mixture in the glass bowl. Use the toothbrush as normal to brush your teeth. Leave the paste for 5 minutes and rinse your mouth.

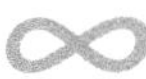

Take a piece of the inside of the banana peel and gently rub around on your teeth for about 2-4 minutes. Leave it for another 5 minutes and rinse your mouth.

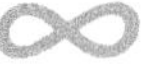

3 tablets of activated charcoal (you can buy at any pharmacy)

Mince them into powder in a glass bowl. You can add a bit of water. Dip your toothbrush into it and brush your teeth. Leave for 5 minutes and then rinse your mouth.

Toothpaste

1 teaspoon coconut Oil

½ teaspoon baking soda

Mix the mixture in a small container and apply on a toothbrush. Brush your teeth as normal. Rinse afterward.

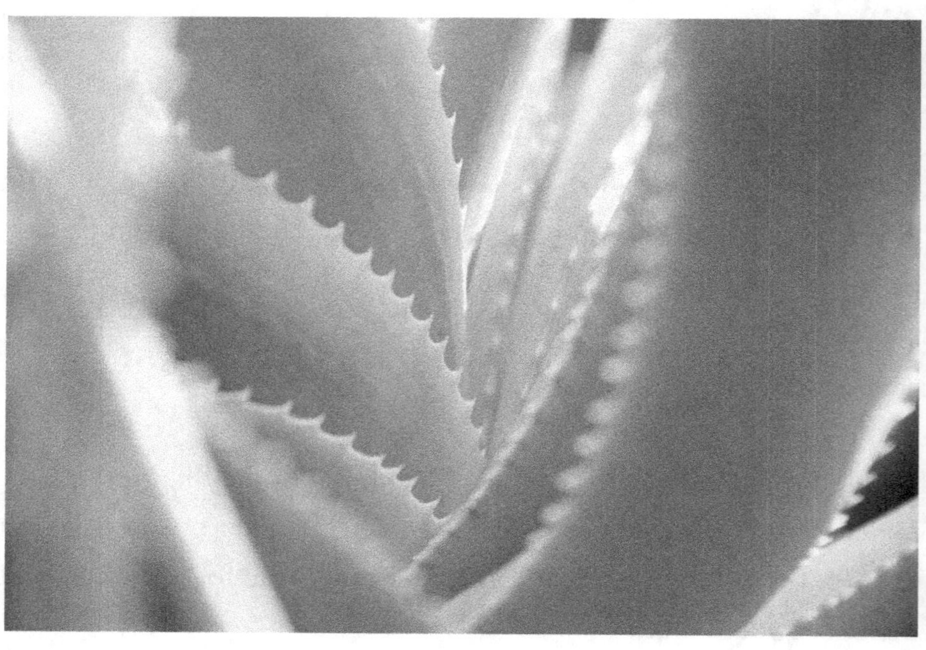

Removing Plaque / Tartar from Teeth

1 glass water

30 g (1.05 oz) walnut shells

Put ingredients in a cooking pot and cook. Cook the walnut shells with water on high heat till it boils and then reduce the heat to low. Cook for about 15-20 min. Leave it on the side. When the mixtures cools down, take a toothbrush and brush your teeth with the solution in a circular motion for about 5 minutes. Repeat this procedure every day for 3-5 days in the morning, mid-afternoon and evening.

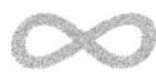

4 tablespoons basswood (could be in tea bags too)

4 tablespoons sunflower seeds

1 L (34 oz) water

Put ingredients into a cooking pot and cook. Cook them on high heat till it boils and then reduce the heat to low. Cook for about 30 min. Leave it on the side. When the mixtures cools down, take a toothbrush and brush your teeth with the solution in a circular motion for about 5 minutes. Repeat this procedure every day for 3-5 days in the morning, mid-afternoon and evening.

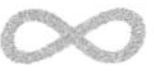

Meg Gordon

GLYCERINE, U. S. P.
CHAS. W. KING
PURE GLYCERINE, U. S. P.
CHAS. W. KING
REGISTERED PHARMACIST
CHICOPEE FALLS, MASS
SPRINGFIELD, MASS

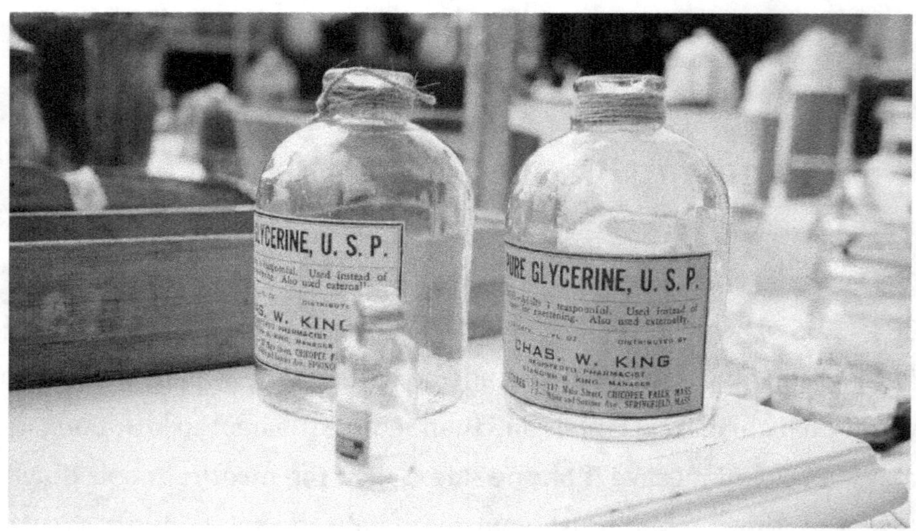